MICRO

HABITS

Small Changes – Big Results

Ron Kness

Published by:

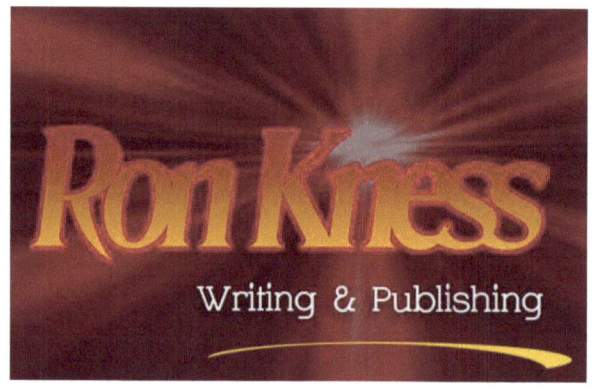

Ron Kness

San Tan Valley

United States of America

ISBN: 9781082071041

Table of Contents

Introduction

Want to change your life? You're fed up with being who you are and can't even see clearly who you want to be. You've crashed and burned too many times before.

Now here you are at a crossroads: do you try one last time, or give up before you even start?

Thankfully, giving up doesn't have to be an option. You can be a better, stronger, more confident version of yourself, and this time you're guaranteed not to fail.

That's because this time you're going to build **micro-habits**. These tiny changes are about to give you some pretty huge results. Part of your previous failures might have been trying to make too many big changes all at once.

Micro-habits are what they sound like – they're small actions that you do on a regular basis until they become a habit. Incremental change has been proven to work, over and over, in a variety of ways. What makes micro-habits so exciting is that they really are tiny. By embracing them, you're not indulging in those grand sweeping gestures that caused you to crash and burn before.

In this book, you're going to first learn the value of incremental change. Then once you understand what a micro-habit is, you'll get a chance to explore a couple dozen that you can start implementing in your life today!

This book will start you off with a variety of suggestions that pertain to Health, Financial Wellness, your Family Life, Career, and even Social Skills.

So, get ready to change your life. You're about to discover a brand new you.

Why Incremental Change?

The phrase "incremental change" might not be familiar to you, but I guarantee that the effects of it are.

Simply put - incremental changes are small shifts over a long period of time.

If you think about the Grand Canyon, you can very easily see the effects of incremental change over a period of thousands and thousands of years.

The tiny erosions of wind and water that carved the Grand Canyon were so minute you could never see the effects of it on a day to day basis. In fact, the Canyon is still changing today. If you visited it thirty years ago and then came back and visited it today, you wouldn't see the same Canyon exactly. But you'd never know it, even if you stood in the exact same spot where you took a picture on that trip thirty years ago and took a picture there now.

In people, incremental change is likewise very gradual. Unless you have several medical issues, you didn't wake up fifty pounds overweight one day, nor did your grandfather acquire those heavy lines etched into his face in the course of an afternoon.

These changes happened over time.

When carving canyons or gaining weight, while the changes themselves were slow and almost entirely unseen, the results are large enough to be visible to those around us. No one can dispute Grandpa's wrinkles any more than they can dispute the depth of the Grand Canyon. This is what makes incremental change so absolutely astonishing in its power.

By focusing on micro-habits, you're going to harness the power of incremental change. By focusing on these tiny actions acted out over time, that are so small that they seem almost unnoticeable to the casual observer, your life is going to change in *great big exciting ways.*

How awesome is that?

Before we begin, let's take just a moment to discuss why using incremental change is so much better than just revamping your entire life all at once.

They are easier to start

Often, the reason we have such a hard time making changes in our lives is that we just don't know where to begin. The whole process seems so daunting and overwhelming. With micro-habits, the difficulty is removed. When you're only changing one very small thing, it barely feels like a change at all. In fact, it can be kind of fun trying out an incremental change just to see what kind of results you get.

They are easier to sustain

While big changes tend to get real old real fast (like changing from a diet full of processed foods over to something Keto or Paleo), micro-changes (like adding a vegetable to every meal) never feel hard at all. The simplicity of incremental change carries momentum all on its own.

The things that burn you out about the old way aren't even an issue in the world of incremental change. You keep going with them, long after you've quit on the big, heavy resolution. This sustainability is what leads to consistently building healthier habits.

They are fairly painless

The big changes are sometimes so sweeping that they can actually hurt. Imagine throwing out every piece of unhealthy food in your kitchen. Then imagine standing there trying to figure out what to eat.

With that kind of sweeping change, if you ended up in tears, it wouldn't be entirely unexpected. After all, you've just lost everything that you *liked* to eat.

The nice thing about micro-habits is that the change is in increments ... small increments. So, if you're working to change your diet, you're only changing out one food perhaps – like giving up soda – while still enjoying the things you usually enjoy.

Chances are you're not going to miss the soda so much if you don't also cut out the chips, cookies, candy, and everything else unhealthy all at once. That makes this kind of change easier to take in the long run.

Also, by making little changes, you're giving yourself time to discover things about you that you never knew before, things that you *like*. So even if you wind up giving up all that junk food, it's ok, because in the process you found that you really love to eat fresh fruit too.

They use less energy

Those great big changes are only going to wear you out. It's like going for a full-fledged workout when you typically rarely leave the couch. Your body certainly isn't ready for that kind of work, and the whole process (finding workout clothes and equipment, going to the gym, knowing what machine to use and how long, and for how many reps) can be pretty daunting.

Micro-habits encourage you to take things slow, leaving you with more energy for the rest of your day. So instead of worrying about all that time at the gym, maybe you're just deciding to take the stairs at work or to park further away from the building, so you get that extra walking in. That bypasses all that energy you'd spend going to and from the gym, and still gives you some exercise you wouldn't normally get.

That's not to say that going to the gym is a bad thing! Even your gym routine could use some additional micro-habits, especially if you're already been going regularly.

So, your usual hour on the treadmill can be easily be adjusted by spending an extra five minutes with weights before calling it a day. You could also commit to trying an additional exercise machine that isn't usually part of your workout.

They keep you motivated

Great big goals can feel a million miles away and easily leave you discouraged.

Micro-habits set smaller goals that are achieved in tiny increments. This means you get to your destination a lot faster, leaving you with a feeling of accomplishment. That feeling helps keep you motivated as you continue to work towards change. Creating micro-habits is a self-sustaining cycle of change and momentum.

While these might not seem like big achievements, the feeling of having done something special is still perfectly valid and will make you feel good about yourself, and what you're doing.

At this point, it's up to you to take that motivation and run with it. Use it to feed the next micro-habit, so that no matter what, you keep moving forward, growing and changing and becoming who you're meant to be. Part of a life-long learning experience.

When you look at all the benefits to be found in micro-habits, you can't help but see that they might be tiny – but they have some big positive value when it comes to making positive change in your life. **Positive change that you can sustain!**

Knowing the value of incremental change, now it's time to run with it.

In the next chapter, you're going to find several suggestions for different micro-habits you can start enjoying right away, along with some tips to help make those habits stick so that you get the full benefit from them.

Micro-habits You Can Start Creating Now

So what are you waiting for? There's no time like the present for getting started on the road to the new you. These changes are so small and easy, you will wonder why you didn't get started earlier!

In the following pages you're going to find a list of tiny habits in various common areas in people's lives, namely:

- Health
- Financial
- Family
- Career
- Social

With each of these habits you'll find a discussion on why this habit works, and some tips for on creating and sustaining that particular habit.

Let's begin!

Health

Because health is the number one thing that people want to change in their lives, we'll begin there.

According to the American Medical Association, as many as 40% of individuals are described as overweight, and 2/3 of those individuals have tried some kind of weight loss / health regimen in the last year.

With so many people concerned with their health, it's no wonder that this is a favorite area to make changes. The good news? Micro-habits work particularly well in this category!

Drink Water

Being chronically dehydrated is such a common thing that it's thought that up to 75% of Americans aren't drinking enough water. But other than being a little dry-mouthed what's the problem? Simply put, dehydration can cause a whole host of health problems that include making it hard to concentrate all the way down to making your heart race. Water is *really* that important!

> ### *What can you do?*
>
> Make a point to drink more water throughout the day. Try setting an alarm on your phone to remind you to stop and grab a drink of water. How much should you have?
>
> Under the old guidelines, it was eight 8-ounce glasses per day. However, the new guidelines recommend taking your weight and dividing that number by 2. That's how many ounces of water you should drink in the course of a day. And it makes more sense since a larger body requires more water.
>
> An added benefit? You'll find you eat less if you're drinking more.

Most of your hunger pangs are actually thirst in disguise. Grab that drink and wait for 20 minutes after drinking and before reaching for a snack; you might find you don't need that snack after all; you were just thirsty. But the two signs are much alike and easily confused.

Walk more

Getting more exercise is integral to good health. But here's where most people go wrong. They hear that you're supposed to walk 10,000 steps in a day to be healthy and suddenly they're trying to step like crazy just to make up the numbers. What many people fail to realize is the steps they take during the day going about their daily business also counts toward the 10,000 step per day goal. Going too hard at the beginning can lead to the classic "crash and burn". While you can't dispute that aerobic exercise is good for you, too much too soon doesn't benefit anyone.

What can you do?

Focus on the micro-habits. Add steps in small ways. Take the parking space further from the door when you're out shopping. Take the stairs instead of the elevator when you get to work. The key here is to be consistent.

Still hung up on that step counter? Then set tiny habits here too. Instead of trying for that 10,000-step goal all at once, set something smaller. Look at how much walking you do usually and challenge yourself to walk a hundred steps further than that each day for the next week. Then build on this number slowly, setting new tiny habits as needed until you're in step with your final goal.

Eat your veggies

While you've probably heard that eating your leafy greens is good for you, do you know why? Veggies are low in the stuff you're trying to avoid – like fat and carbohydrates – and high in the stuff you want – like vitamins and minerals which your body needs to keep running at optimal condition. They're also loaded in fiber, something else we typically don't get enough of.

What can you do?

Try adding a vegetable to your plate at every meal. There're so many great veggies to choose from that you can try a different one every day and not run out of ideas for months. Try cooking them in different ways than you usually do, making a micro-habit of trying out new recipes. You can even simplify things by just committing to eating veggies raw as your afternoon snack.

Don't forget the protein

While veggies are an obvious choice for your good health, did you know that you likewise need protein in your diet as well? In fact, you should be eating protein at every meal. Why? Protein is one of those building blocks for things like bone, muscles, and blood.

But more than that, eating protein is good for your metabolism, especially if you're trying to lose weight. It also helps to keep your blood sugar up (which might be important if you're dropping a lot of carbs for other reasons).

What can you do?

This is a fairly easy tiny habit to build. Simply make a point to add protein at every meal. Or decide to make protein part of your snacking habit by adding nuts or other high protein foods to your repertoire.

Get up and stretch

Most jobs tend toward being fairly sedentary, and while you might thank your lucky stars that you don't have a job that keeps you on your feet all day, you're not doing your body any favors by sitting.

In fact, long periods of time spent at your desk are hard on your body, making you prone to obesity, heart disease, diabetes, and other various problems. You really do need to get up and move around once in a while.

What can you do?

Again, here's one of those perfect opportunities to grab your timer. Make a point to get up and stretch every hour. Or find a Micro Routine of stretches you can do at your desk. Doing a search online will show you a whole slew of stretches that will help you to get in motion quickly and easily. As an added bonus, regular stretching will help with any new exercise habits you create.

Get adequate sleep

According to the CDC, 1 in 3 people aren't getting enough sleep at night. There is even some thought that the actual number might be higher. We all know we feel better with enough rest, but it can be more important than just how we feel.

Shortchanging yourself will make you tired the next day, and is hard on your body as well, making you more susceptible to illness, and even straining things like your heart.

What can you do?

Set a tiny habit that helps you set up for a good night's sleep. Remove your phone from your bedroom at night. Set a bedtime goal of lights out by a certain time.

Or establish a habit of reading or doing something equally relaxing before bed that helps the mind to shut down. Just remember to avoid blue light emitting devices like e-readers, smartphones, etc. Your body needs 7 – 9 hours of sleep at night; it's up to you to make sure you get it.

Financial

Sixty-three percent of Americans are in debt of some kind, and 14.5% of Americans are living below the poverty line. Those kinds of numbers make it very clear that there's a lot of people who aren't happy with their financial status and would like to make some serious changes when it comes to cash flow.

Tiny habits can help here too, in a variety of ways.

Educate yourself

When trying to keep on track financially, half the battle is having a good sense of how budgeting, finances, long-range planning, and economics works. Taking the time to educate yourself helps you to make wiser decisions in regard to your financial future. Thankfully there are lots of great resources out there (from books to blogs to podcasts) that are full of great information to help you get your financial future on track.

What can you do?

Make a goal to read a page of a book every day. Or listen to a podcast on your daily commute. Or make a point to subscribe to blogs that you find inspirational or helpful and then create the micro-habit of reading them whenever you have the chance. **Pro tip:** Audiobooks are great for long drives or commutes.

Buy quality

It's so easy to get caught up in the idea that buying cheap saves you money. But does it really? That coat you got at the discount store might save you a few dollars now, but will it last more than one winter? Or worse, if the shoddy zipper breaks you might be out of luck because you don't have the cash to buy another one. When buying quality, you save money in the long run.

What can you do?

Create micro-habits that help keep you informed. Try spending a few minutes before any major purchase to check ratings and reviews online to see if the quality is what you're hoping for.

Become familiar with the earmarks of quality by asking questions and doing your research. While these might not seem like micro-habits at first glance, consistently asking questions before any major purchase is exactly that – a small habit designed to make you pause and make sure you're getting the best quality *and* that you're getting that quality for the best price.

Watch your spending

It's so easy to spend far more than you intend. Even those of us who set the most detailed budgets, might end up scrambling at the end of the month. On top of that, setting budgets is typically overwhelming. This is where tiny habits come into play.

What can you do?

Carry a small notebook to jot down expenses so that you're more aware of where your money goes (you can also use a notes app on your phone).

Create a micro-habit where you ask yourself "Do I need that" every single time before you actually spend the money. Or before hitting the cash register at the grocery store, remove three superfluous items from your cart.

For bigger purchases try creating a habit of a 24-hour rule, meaning you must sleep on it before making a final decision.

Create savings

Putting money away for the future sounds like a pipe dream, especially when most people struggle to make ends meet in the first place.

But think about it. What if you actually had a cushion for that car emergency? Or could actually afford to go on vacation once in a while? It might not seem possible now, but a couple of micro-habits could make it a reality.

What can you do?

Micro-habits really show their stuff in this category because there are so many ways to save. Here are just a few easy ones...

- Start a change jar for the loose coins in your pockets at the end of the day.
- Stick $5 or $10 in an envelope at the end of the week and put that away in a special place to have for something special at the end of the year.
- Give up something that's non-essential that you tend to spend money on daily (like that fancy coffee) and then put the money you'd spend on that item in your savings account instead.

Little tiny savings like this add up very quickly. You'd be surprised at how much money you can save by the end of the year. It might not change your life, but it will certainly make for a nice treat.

Family

Our relationships within our families can be especially tricky.

Most people, when asked, would tell you that they don't feel like they spend enough time with their families. What's worse is that even when they do have that time to spend, they feel distant and disconnected.

It's these feelings that lead to a breakdown in the family structure and can lead to estranged relationships and even divorce. Given how important our families are in our lives, it's good to know that tiny habits can strengthen even these relationships and help instigate positive change where it's needed the most.

Teach gratitude

A grateful heart tends to be a heart that's at peace with the world around them. By teaching your kids about gratitude early on you help to instill values in them that they'll carry with them for the rest of their lives.

A spirit of gratitude will always know contentment and enjoy better family relationships than those who are dissatisfied.

What can you do?

As far as micro-habits are concerned, teach your kids from early on to start their day by saying something that they're thankful for before they even get out of bed. This is such a small thing but starts the day in such a positive way. Or try a family gratitude journal where any family member can record something that they're grateful for. Then make it a micro-habit to share that journal periodically with the rest of the family.

Build family habits

Some habits just need to be built right into your family. Things like always saying "please" and "thank you" for example. We're used to thinking of these things as family rules because they help everyone to get along a little bit better. Whatever you call them, these guidelines are very necessary for your family relationships.

What can you do?

Start with your manners. Build the micro-habit of always saying 'please' and then add in another for 'thank you' when you have that one down. Each family rule should be a tiny habit all by itself and should build on the others to make for a cohesive family unit that works and plays well together.

Create time together

As the saying goes, 'the family that plays together, stays together.'

How true that is might be up for debate, but there have been plenty of studies that show the benefit of kids sitting down at the dinner table with their parents. And even when you're talking about extended family members, spending actual time together is the surest way to maintain healthy bonds.

What can you do?

Since we're only looking at micro-habits, we're not looking for big sweeping changes designed to shift the entire family dynamic.

Instead focus on the small stuff: Make a point to have at least one meal with everyone together at the table once a week. Try creating a family game night or take up another family hobby like hiking. Because every family is different, it's up to you to find the small things that will make the biggest differences.

Maybe for you, that means never missing a soccer game. For someone else, it might be a Saturday movie night.

Communicate more

How can you possibly expect to get along with someone that you never even talk to? Or worse, to be understood by someone who would rather argue than listen to what you have to say?

Communication is so important to the family dynamic that it gets its own discussion here. If communication breaks down, so does the family. That's why it's so important to not only speak your piece but to listen when others speak theirs.

What can you do?

Micro-habits here might involve checking in with the other family members n a regular basis. Maybe that means calling your mom once a week. Or making a point to follow your sister on social media.

At home, you want to encourage communication within your own family, especially with your spouse, at every opportunity. Try a 5-minute rule where each spouse gets five minutes to talk about their day every night while the other listens. Then try switching it up so that the other listens while the other spouse speaks. To further the marriage relationship, you also might try instituting a habit of putting love notes where the other will see them. Or calling during the occasional lunch hour to check in and chat about your day.

With your kids, try building a micro-habit of asking your child what they liked best about the day as part of the bedtime routine and then really listen when they answer. Put notes in their lunches.

Or try a mall date with your teen once a month where you combine shopping with a long heart-to-heart over lunch.

Career

According to Gallup Polls, 85% of people hate their jobs. ...Yikes!

Given how much time you spend each week working, this is a serious problem. A dislike of your job or a workplace that's unpleasant can lead to high-stress levels which in turn impact your health negatively.

Incremental change has the solution you need to turn this aspect of your life around. Wouldn't you rather be in the 15% who love what they do? You'd be surprised how much of success lies in your attitude.

Pay attention to ideas
Writing down ideas as they come to you, means you are less likely to miss opportunities in the workplace.

But did you know that by stopping to write down ideas every day you train yourself to become more creative and to think outside the box? Employees who can think on their feet and come up with alternative solutions are much sought after in the workplace and have more opportunity for advancement.

What can you do?

Build a micro-habit of writing down ideas every day.

Some say to write down 10 new ideas every morning, but if that number feels daunting then reduce it to something you're more comfortable with. After all, you're trying to set micro-habits here!

Other small behaviors you can set? Always carry a notebook to write down ideas as they come to you. Or when watching TV and seeing characters confronted with a problem, pause the show and brainstorm how you would solve it. Then hit play and see how close you came to their solution.

Single-task

As much as we hate to admit it, it's been proven time, and again that multitasking *simply doesn't work.*

We not only get less done when we're trying to do several things at once, but we actually reduce our IQ by several points when we do.

What can you do?

Design a micro-habit to cut out distractions. Turn off your phone while working. Or make a point to not look at email as it comes in. Create habits that enable you to find and keep your focus. Leverage whatever tools necessary to keep you on track.

Optimize your work time

Much like the last item on this list, you get more done when you're focused. But this time, you want to concentrate on your work schedule itself. How do you make the most of your time at work and still get done what you need to?

What can you do?

Start by knowing when you're most productive. If you're sharpest when you first get to work, then create tiny habits that remind you to do the big projects first.

For that matter, micro-habits work really well with schedules, so think about using your phone to set blocks of work time using the Pomodoro technique.

Or set reminders on your phone to get up and stretch periodically, so that your mind stays alert and you don't drag quite so much in the afternoon.

Also, think about small habits that keep your workspace neat and tidy, so you can always find what you need when you need it.

Re-assess your goals

By keeping your eye on the prize, you know if you're actually working toward something – or allowing yourself to get derailed completely.

In order to do that, you need to revisit these goals every so often. Look at what you've accomplished and asked yourself what you want to accomplish next. Make sure every goal is S.M.A.R.T.: specific, measurable, attainable, relevant, and time-bound.

What can you do?

Set micro-habits to check in with yourself by setting a date on the calendar once a month to re-assess. Or use an app to track progress on projects.

Again, these are small habits, so you're not looking at the goals you're setting, which are big picture things, but at the small things – the check-ins, the progress you're making today, and the questions you need to ask yourself to see if you're still on task.

Seize Opportunities

Things will come up in your workplace that will give you a chance at advancement, or at the very least to come into the boss's line of sight. The more opportunities you find, the more you'll find room for advancement.

What can you do?

Keep an ear to the ground. Micro-habits here include paying attention to the company newsletter, the bulletin board, or wherever they post notices. Make a point to check the news daily. You never know what might come up.

Outside of your workplace, make a tiny goal to spend a few minutes on LinkedIn or other professional sites to network. Don't worry about loyalty, use these sites to stay on the lookout for new job opportunities.
if you're seriously thinking about changing jobs, maybe your micro-goal will be to spend time learning a new skill that might come in handy later.

Social

Your social life is just as important as the other topics here. Having real relationships with people you can count on is an integral part of a happy life.

Being able to build better relationships and be more confident through the use of micro-habits is something you should definitely be striving for. How do you do that?

Reach out to others

It's impossible to have a social life if you're not...well...*social*.

In order to solve that most basic of problems, you're going to have to interact with people at some point. Reaching out should be fairly obvious. Establishing good micro-habits here will help to make that easier.

What can you do?

A simple micro-habit could be setting a day of the week to call an old friend. Or making a point to spend a little time on social media to re-connect with people that you haven't seen for a while.

What about a setting up a once a week casual get-together with co-workers after work? None of these should be big complicated things. Just start with showing up, saying hi and letting the interactions flow from there.

Schedule time out for yourself

Make time spent with friends something that's really intentional by putting your get-togethers on the calendar where nothing else can interfere with that time.

By scheduling this time you're telling yourself that this is important and not to be missed. You are committed to not staying home and getting out into the world.

What can you do?

In the world of micro-habits, this one doesn't have to be hard. Maybe it's as simple as making it a point to get out at least once a week with friends.

Again, you're looking at small changes in your life, so this doesn't have to involve planning a big gala party, but just something small and casual. Grab a friend and catch a movie. Go to a bar. Sing karaoke. Tailor this one to your own likes and dislikes.

Can't find anyone to go with? Then go by yourself. The point is you're making an effort to get out. Who knows, you might meet someone wherever you wind up.

Catch a bite with friends

One of the most casual ways to socialize is to ask someone out for coffee or for a quick meal. Food makes social gatherings easy because it gives you something to do while hanging out (eating) and also gives you something to talk about (the food/service/restaurant).

What can you do?

A simple and easy habit to start is just reaching out to friends and coworkers to see if they'd like to grab a bite to eat.

What about pulling together people from work who go out to lunch together at least once a week? Or make a point to meet a friend for coffee on the weekends.

Again, this is a small habit, so you don't have to go crazy here. The point is getting out and making sure that you have company for this adventure.

Join a group
Sometimes the best way to socialize is to spend time with people who enjoy the same things you do.
Joining a church, club, community organization, book club, or political party are all ways to get out and meet people with like interests.

The nice thing is that you can find groups for anything from Art Appreciation to Yoga, so it's pretty easy to find something that interests you where you can meet like-minded people.

What can you do?

Micro-habits here involve making a regular commitment to spend time with a certain group of people.

It might be that your habit is to go to church every Sunday. Or to visit the book club at the library that meets once a week.

Other habits might involve volunteering for a political organization or at an animal shelter. The main thing is to be consistent. It's hard to form friendships if you're just dipping in and out of various groups. Choose something that interests you and create a micro-habit of attending weekly. Commit for at least a month to give the group/activity a fair chance.

Say 'yes.'

While many self-help books warn you repeatedly to protect your best interests by knowing when to say 'no' – when it comes to expanding your social horizons the rules change.

In fact, you can't get anywhere unless you find the ability to say 'yes' once in a while. This means accepting that invitation to lunch or agreeing to go with to the ball game next Saturday. You don't have to say 'yes' to things you have absolutely no interest in, but don't be so quick to say 'no' right off the bat.

What can you do?

Your micro-habit here should be as simple as "saying yes to social invitations that involve certain people or situations."

By making a 'yes' response habitual, you open yourself up to opportunity and new situations. What's more, you're giving yourself the chance to know someone a little better.

***

While looking for ways to improve yourself, keep in mind that the ideas presented in this book are just that – ideas. Consider these micro-habits listed as jumping off points. After all, no one knows you better than you.

Think about what your personal needs are, and how you can better meet those needs. Then take those big ideas and break them down into smaller ones in order to set in place the incremental change needed to succeed.

The key here is to keep the changes small so that you have a better chance for success.

Lastly, keep in mind that you didn't get where you are today overnight. So too, you can't fix everything in the course of a single day. Don't overwhelm yourself with a whole slew of micro-habits all at once. Pick a few to focus on, with the realization that you can always go back later and add more into your routine.

In the end, all you need to realize is that adopting micro-habits will change your life. Once you try them, you'll never be the same person again.

Conclusion

Who knew that such tiny habits could have such a big impact on every aspect of your life?

By embracing incremental change, you'll find that you are making progress on your desired changes, almost without effort!

You will also find that you feel healthier and happier than ever before. You'll feel motivated and really have the energy to embrace this brand new you.

Remember, micro-habits work in multiple aspects of your life:

- Health
- Financial
- Family
- Career
- Social

When you make a list of things that you want to change in your life, remember to think small. Determine the micro-habits that will get you where you want to go.

Then be consistent and allow these changes to become a habit, a way of life. And don't give up on a micro-change. Remember it takes between 21 and 30 days for a change to become a habit.

Get ready to embrace the new you that's waiting just around the corner.

How exciting is that?

The Workbook

If you are interested in getting more out of this book and using a guided strategy to guide you into making little changes to your habits that yield big results, consider adding this workbook to your micro-habit change plan.

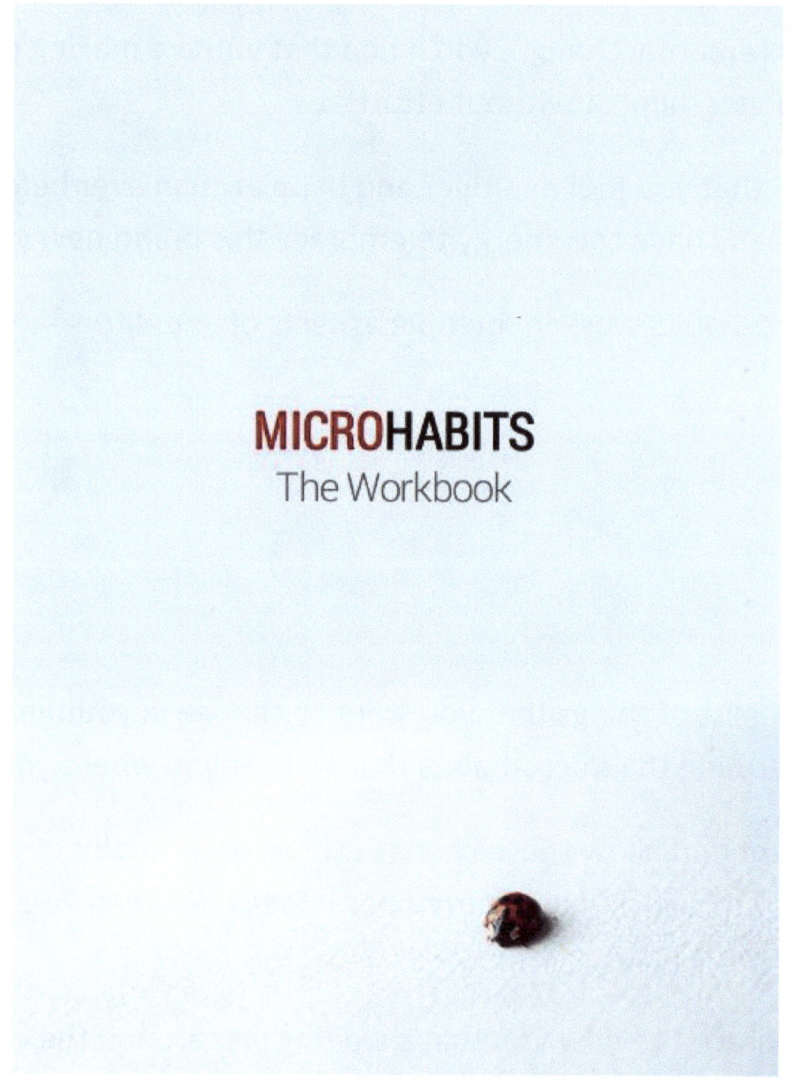

https://www.paypal.com/cgi-bin/webscr?cmd=_s-xclick&hosted_button_id=5RX2WLRAY2RUY

About the Author

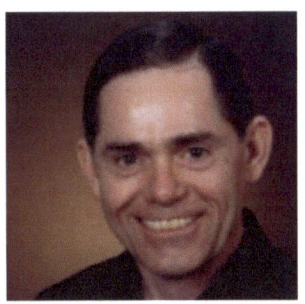

I have published numerous books on Amazon for Kindle and other publishing platforms. Both in electronic and POD formats.

While most of my books are on health and fitness in general, my topics of interest are leaning more toward aging baby boomers and the older population.

Besides my own writing, I also ghostwrite ebooks, books, reports, articles, blogs and do Kindle conversions for clients on a variety of topics. For a complete list of books, go to https://www.amazon.com/Ron-Kness/e/B0072M6PYO.

Today my wife and I are retired from our careers and live in San Tan Valley, AZ. I now write as a retirement business where you'll find me happily sitting in my office typing away on my laptop as I work on my next book or ghostwriting project . . . that is if we are not traveling on a cruise ship - our new-found mode of travel.

www.ingramcontent.com/pod-product-compliance
Lightning Source LLC
Chambersburg PA
CBHW041826280526
45792CB00006B/2010

* 9 7 8 1 0 8 2 0 7 1 0 4 1 *